BENEFITS OF
ARGAN OIL

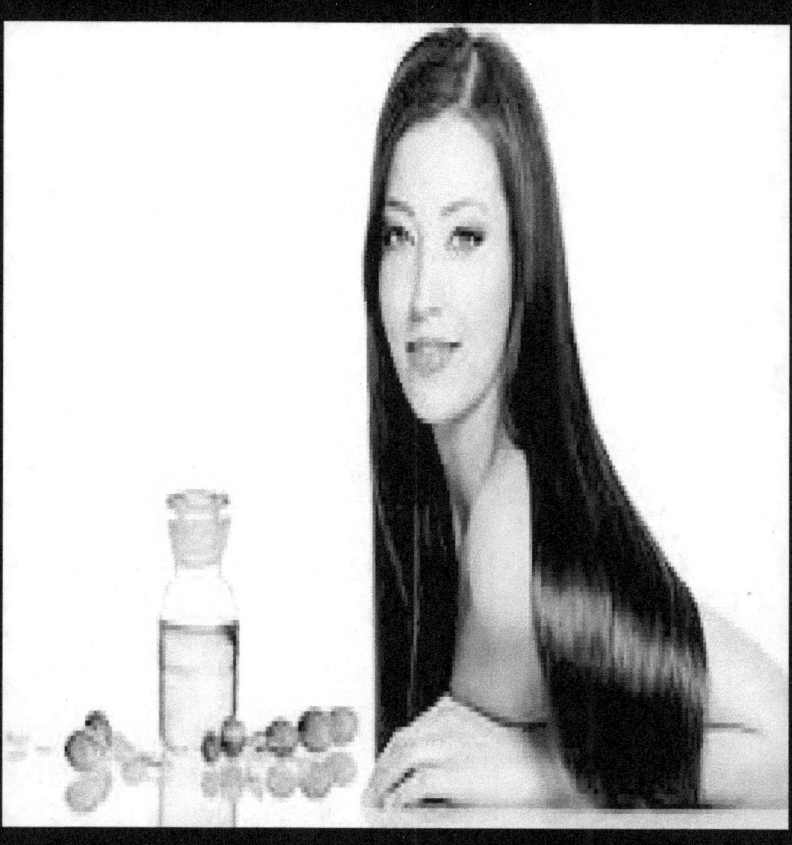

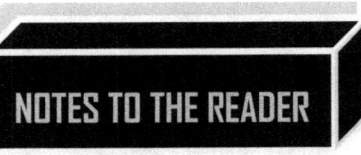

NOTES TO THE READER

While the authors of this book have made reasonable efforts to ensure the accuracy and timeliness of the information contained herein, the author and publisher assume no liability with respect to loss or damage caused, or alleged to be caused, by any reliance on any information contained herein and disclaim any and all warranties, expressed or implied, as to the accuracy or reliability of said information. The authors make no representations or warranties with respect to the accuracy or completeness of the contents of this work and specifically disclaim all warranties. The advice and strategies contained herein may not be suitable for every situation. It is the complete responsibility of the reader to ensure they are adhering to all local, regional and national laws. This publication is designed to provide accurate and authoritative information in regard to the subject matter covered.

TABLE OF CONTENTS

WHAT IS ARGAN OIL?

Argan oil is a plant oil created from the parts of the argan tree (Argania spinosa L.) that is endemic to Morocco. In Morocco, argan oil is utilized to dunk bread in at breakfast or to sprinkle on couscous or pasta. It is additionally utilized for corrective purposes.

The product of the argan tree is little, and round, oval, or cone like. A thick peel covers the beefy mash. The mash encompasses a hard-shelled nut that speaks to around 25% of the heaviness of the new organic product.

The nut contains one to three oil-rich argan pieces. Extraction yields from 30% to half of the oil in the parts, contingent upon the extraction strategy.

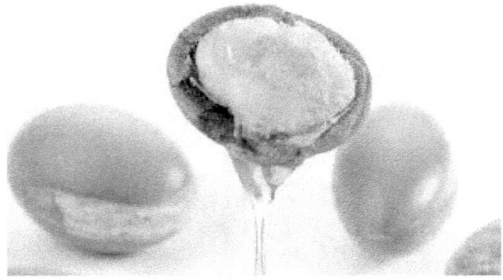

Extraction is vital to the creation procedure. To extricate the parts, laborers first dry argan natural product in the outside and after that evacuates the beefy mash. A few makers evacuate the substance mechanically without drying the organic product. Moroccans for the most part utilize the tissue as creature encourage.

The following stage includes popping the argan nut to acquire the argan parts. Endeavours to automate this procedure have been unsuccessful, so specialists still do it by hand, making it a tedious, work concentrated process. Berber ladies frequently take part in this challenging errand.

Laborers tenderly dish portions they will use to make culinary argan oil. After the argan parts cool, laborers crush and squeeze them. The chestnut shaded pound ousts unadulterated, unfiltered argan oil. At last, they empty unfiltered argan oil into vessels. The rest of the squeeze cake is protein-rich and much of the time utilized as cows bolster.

Restorative argan oil is delivered indistinguishably, however the argan bits are not broiled to dodge a too much nutty aroma.

The emptied argan oil is left to rest around two weeks with the goal that solids suspended in the argan oil settle to the base, making characteristic silt. The clearer argan oil is further separated, contingent upon the required clarity and immaculateness. Unadulterated argan oil may contain some dregs. This is a characteristic part of the generation procedure and does not influence quality.

Culinary argan oil (argan sustenance oil) is utilized for plunging bread, on couscous, plates of mixed greens and comparative employments. Amlou, a thick cocoa glue with a consistency like nutty spread, is delivered by pounding cooked almond and argan oil utilizing stones, blended with nectar and is utilized locally as a bread plunge.

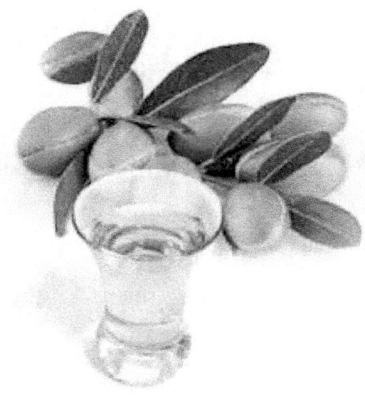

Different claims about the helpful consequences for wellbeing because of the utilization of argan oil have been made. An examination article distributed in 2010 found that argan oil contained more elevated amounts than different oils of γ-Tocopherol, which has solid chemo preventive and mitigating properties

Moroccans customarily utilize un-cooked Argan oil to treat skin illnesses, and as restorative oil for skin and hair:

"In beauty care products, Argan oil is upheld as saturating oil, against skin inflammation vulgaris and chipping of the skin, and in addition for "feeding" the hair. This oil has likewise [sic] therapeutic uses against stiffness and the mending of blazes. Remotely, Argan oil is utilized for hair as brilliantine, to strengthen and in the treatment of wrinkled or layered dry skin."

Argan oil has turned out to be progressively prominent for corrective utilize. The quantity of individual care items on the US showcase with Argan oil as a fixing expanded from only two in 2007 to more than 100 by 2011. It is here and there blended with pomegranate seed oil because of its antioxidant benefits, with merchants advancing this mix as a holding nothing back one serum both for skin and hair. Argan oil is likewise sold without added substances as a characteristic skincare and hair mind item.

The expanding ubiquity of Argan oil has incited the Moroccan government to get ready for expanded creation, with their point being to build yearly generation from around 2,500 to 4,000 tons by 2020.

The argan tree gives sustenance, haven and insurance from desertification. The trees' profound roots forestall leave infringement. The covering of argan trees likewise gives shade to other horticultural items, and the leaves and natural product give bolster to creatures.

The argan tree additionally scenes solidness, counteracting soil disintegration, giving shade to pasture grasses, and renewing aquifers.

Creating argan oil has shielded argan trees from being chopped down. What's more, recovery of the Arganeraie has likewise been done: in 2009 an operation to plant 4,300 argan plants was propelled in Meskala in the region of Essaouira.

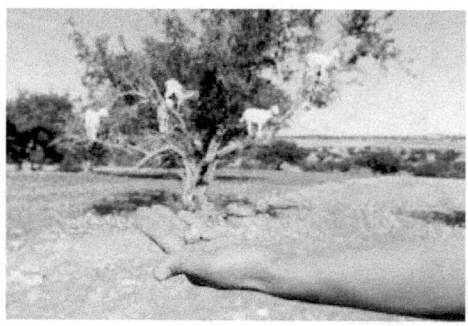

The Réseau des Associations de la Réserve de Biosphère Arganeraie (Network of Associations of the Argan Biosphere Reserve, RARBA) was established in 2002 with the point of guaranteeing manageable advancement in the Arganeraie.

RARBA has been included with a few noteworthy undertakings, including the Moroccan national antidesertification (Program National de Lutte contre la desertification, PAN/LCD). The venture included nearby populaces and encouraged with enhancements to fundamental foundation, administration of common assets, income creating exercises (counting argan oil generation), limit support, and others.

The generation of argan oil has dependably had a financial capacity. At present, argan oil creation bolsters around 2.2 million individuals in the primary argan oil-delivering district, the Arganeraie.

A significant part of the argan oil delivered today is made by some of ladies' co-agents. Co-supported by the Social Development Agency with the support of the European Union, the Union des Cooperatives des Femmes de l'Arganeraie is the biggest union of argan oil co-agents in Morocco. It includes 22 co-agents that are found in different parts of the district (e.g., Coopérative Al Amal, Coopérative Amalou N'Touyag, Coopérative Tissaliwine, Coopérative ArganSense, and Coopérative Maouriga).

Work in the co-agents furnishes ladies with a pay, which numerous have used to store instruction for themselves or their kids. It has additionally furnished them with a level of self-governance in a generally male-ruled society and has helped numerous turned out to be more mindful of their rights.

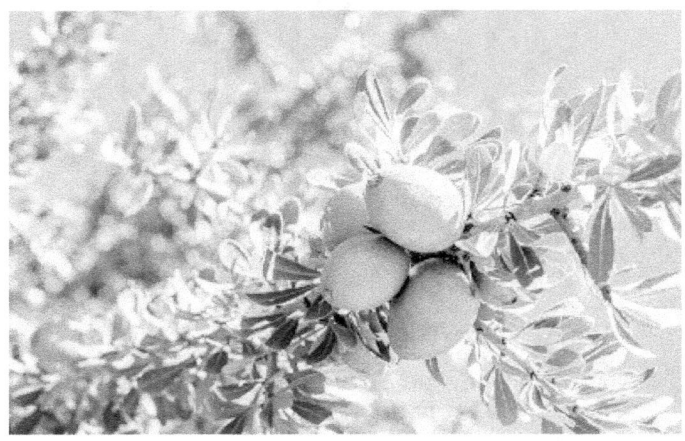

The achievement of the argan co-agents has additionally empowered different makers of farming items to receive the co-agent show. The foundation of the co-agents has been helped by support from inside Morocco, prominently the Fondation Mohamed VI pour la Recherche et la Sauvegarde de l'Arganier (Mohammed VI Foundation for Research and Protection of the Argan Tree), and from worldwide associations, including Canada's International Development Research Center and the European Commission.

Argan oil comes from the fruit of the argan tree, which is endemic to Morocco. This extremely rare oil is traditionally produced by hand and is known to have a number of beneficial properties relating to skin care. The benefits of argan oil are innumerable and proven by scientific research which makes it much sought after. Let's take a quick look at some of its major benefits:

SIMPLE BEAUTY USES FOR ORGANIC ARGAN OIL

Argan oil is created from an Argan nut originating from Argan tree, which just develops in Southwestern Morocco.

Nearby Berber ladies work in reasonable exchange cooperatives where they hand-open the argan nuts in the middle of two stones, a system they've utilized for quite a long time. Rather than being put through a machine, the crude argan bits are hand-extricated from the hard shell, hand-ground in a stone processor, hand-massaged for a considerable length of time and first cool squeezed into the oil. It takes one lady three days to make only one liter of oil. This is the reason argan oil is so important.

In 1998, the Argan timberland in Morocco was assigned an UNESCO secured biosphere so argan oil is reasonable.

In the event that you need to de-mess your bureau and disentangle your excellence schedule, argan oil can turn into your go-to magnificence remedy from go to toe. It's stuffed with crucial unsaturated fats, hostile to oxidants, vitamins and minerals that advance your general wellbeing by saturating, softening and shielding your face and hair from sun harm – without unsafe poisons and Parabens.

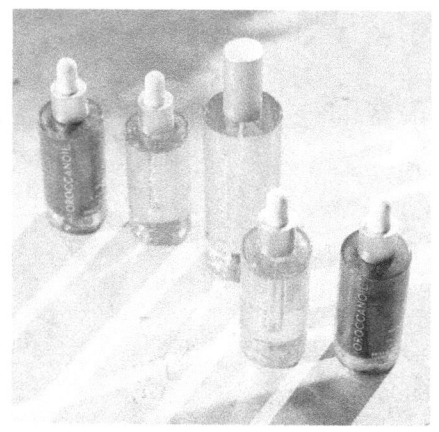

1. Confront cream

In the wake of purifying morning as well as night, back rub a couple drops of argan oil straightforwardly onto your face and neck. Since argan is viewed as a dry oil, it retains rapidly and is not oily. On the off chance that you need to utilize it as a serum, apply your night cream after the oil retains into the skin.

2. Hydrating toner

Include a couple drops of argan oil to your most loved facial toner to hydrate and tone all the while. You can make your own toner by including a couple drops of argan oil to Rose or Orange Blossom water.

3. Reviving and lighting up face cover

Include a couple drops of argan oil to your locally acquired cover. On the other hand, make your own cover by blending 1 tablespoon of lemon juice, 3 teaspoons of Greek-style yogurt, 1 tablespoon of nectar and 3 drops of argan oil in a bowl. Apply on a spotless, dry face and leave on for 10 minutes. Flush off with warm water.

4. Shedding lip scour and lotion

To smooth and saturate your lips, include a couple drops of argan oil and vanilla concentrate to fine chestnut sugar. Daintily knead into lips utilizing roundabout movement and flush off.

5. Confront sparkle

Include a drop or two of argan oil to your establishment, bronzer or tinted cream for a dewy, brilliant shine.

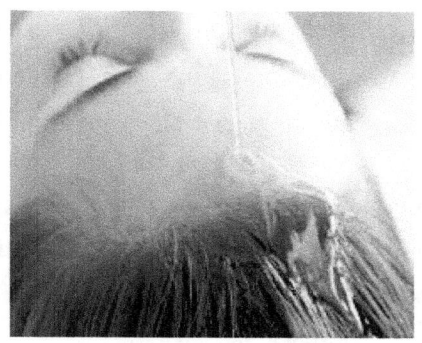

6. Leave-on conditioner

After the shower, while your hair is still wet, include a couple drops of argan oil to your hair, closures and scalp to hydrate and saturate. It's particularly supporting if your hair is dry from everyday utilization of a blow dryer, straight-iron or hair curler.

7. Hair styling sparkle

At the point when your hair is dry, use as a styling item by including a couple drops of argan oil to the palms of your hand. Rub your hands together and run your fingers through your hair to make sparkle and manageable frizz. You just need a little sum. It keeps going quite a while.

8. Overnight hair treatment

Rub a liberal measure of argan oil into your hair, finishes and scalp. Wrap your hair and abandon it on while you rest. In the morning, wash your hair and you'll have radiant, delicate locks.

9. Fingernail skin and heel conditioner

Knead a couple drops of argan oil into your fingernail skin to mellow, saturate and empower nail development. Use as an overnight treatment to feed broke heels by working a decent sum into your feet and toes. Cover with socks and wake up to supple feet.

The not-so-popular use of oil is of nail care. It is rich in vitamins and mineral those are needed for healthy growth of nails and thus repair brittle nails. The oil also moisturizes and strengthens your nail to make it stronger and shinier.

These are just a small number of uses and benefits of this astonishing natural oil, it's certainly a versatile oil that treats many issues and deals with them very well and the best part is... it is 100% natural and totally chemical free.With so many proven benefits of oil, every bit of its popularity is worth it!

10. Body and shower oil

Include a couple drops of argan oil specifically onto your skin, into the shower or body salve. It's sheltered to use on an infant and to minimize extend blemishes on a pregnant gut as well.

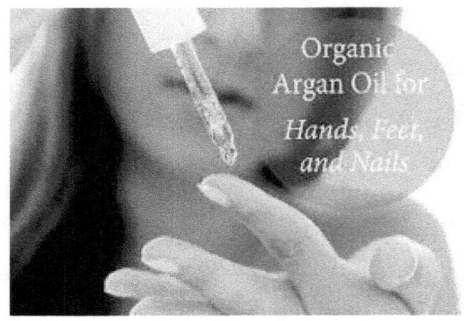

This magical oil is not only beneficial for outward appearance, but, when used in cooking, it can enhance health. Around 70 calories per teaspoon without any trans fat, sodium or cholesterol, Argan oil consumed through diet assists in improving a number of health problems. It is acknowledged to keep blood sugar levels stable. This is key for people with diabetes. Many of those who suffer because of joint inflammation and muscle pain can attain some relief by either consuming Argan oil or by rubbing it onto the affected areas of the body. It increases blood circulation and guards against inflammation related diseases. Long term usage can give a boost to your body's immune system to the point that the risk of a number of types of cancer, like prostate cancer, is decreased.

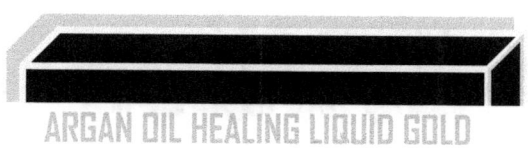

As of late, a mind blowing oil from Morocco called Argan oil (Argania spinosa) has turned out to be such a hot product, to the point that a New York Times publication named it "fluid gold."

Since its fleeting move in fame, the advantages of argan oil have been the subject of various researches contemplates. The demonstrated advantages of this nectar shaded substance with a hazelnut flavor are very noteworthy. As such, studies show that Argan oil can avoid prostate malignancy, bring down cholesterol, and anticipate or turn around different sicknesses.

AT THE POINT WHEN APPLIED TO THE SKIN, PURE ARGAN OIL BENEFITS PROVE TO BE BOTH HEALING AND ANTI-AGING.

The dynamic characteristic fixings in argan oil are amazing, and incorporate...

• Tocopherols

• Squalene

• Carotenes

• Sterols

• Phenolic cancer prevention agents

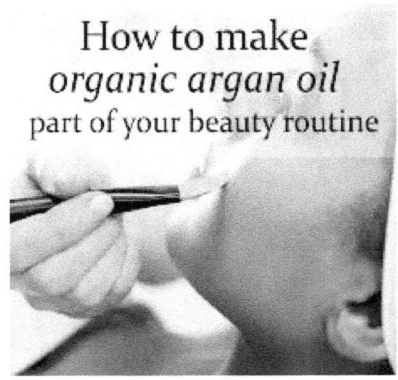

ADVANTAGES OF ARGAN OIL FOR INTERNAL AND EXTERNAL HEALING

There are two evaluations of Argan oil: culinary and corrective. The culinary form possesses a flavor like a smokier sesame oil and is uncommonly useful for your inside organs. The restorative review offers remarkable advantages for the body's biggest organ, the skin.

Unadulterated Argan oil utilized inside has been appeared to battle malignancy, cardiovascular malady, and fiery issue. At the point when connected remotely, it cures everything from scars to diseases to part closures to extend marks.

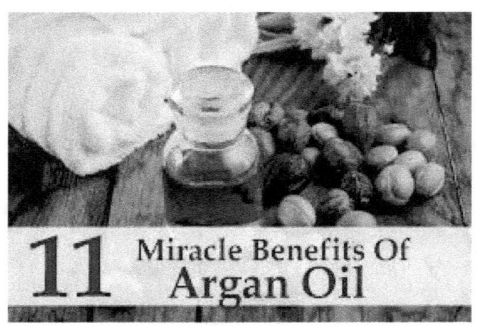

SUPERFOOD, SUPREME

Dr. Philip Steig, Ph.D., M.D., teacher and executive of the Department of Neurological Surgery at Weill Cornell Medical College and Neurosurgeon-in-Chief at New York Presbyterian Hospital, said specialists are hailing the advantages of Argan oil as the most up to date super nourishment.

"As a dependable guideline, around 30% of your eating routine ought to originate from fat," said Steig, "close to ¼ from soaked fats, for example, meat and spread." The rest ought to originate from more beneficial, mono-and polyunsaturated fats.

Set up wellsprings of these sound fats include:

• Nuts

• Fish

• Sesame oil

• Sunflower oil

• Canola oil

• Olive oil

Argan oil out does each and every one of these other nourishment sources.

It contains more beneficial omega 3s than olive oil, more vitamin E than sweet almond oil, and heap growth battling cancer prevention agents, also.

Logical research proposes that culinary Argan oil can help to…

• Lower cholesterol

• Improve dissemination

• Stabilize glucose

• Ease torment from ailment and joint pain

• Strengthen the body's insusceptible framework

• Prevent different sorts of tumor

• Reducing the body's imperviousness to insulin, treating diabetes

• Protecting the body from cardiovascular and fiery infections

Moreover, the oil is delectable. In Morocco, it's eaten with bread, couscous, servings of mixed greens, and then some. To make "Amlou," what might as well be called nutty spread, essentially pound simmered almonds into immaculate Argan oil and appreciate the rich taste of this sound other option to your most loved nut spread.

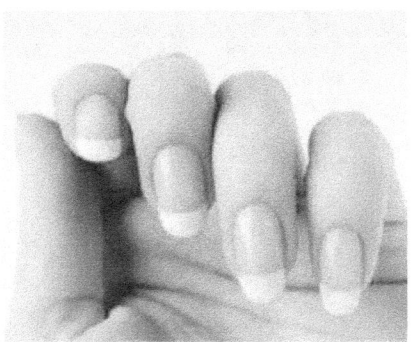

CONVENTIONAL USES OF MOROCCO'S GOLDEN OIL

In Morocco, the main place where the Argan tree is normally found, the oil's astounding remedial properties have been respected for a considerable length of time. In the southern districts of the nation, immaculate Argan oil is praised for everything from mitigating skin redness to curing ailment and the sky is the limit from there.

Customarily, Argan oil has been utilized topically to:

• Protect against and mend skin diseases

• Clear up skin inflammation

• Ease dermatitis

• Hasten recuperation from chicken pox

• Heal breaks and smolders

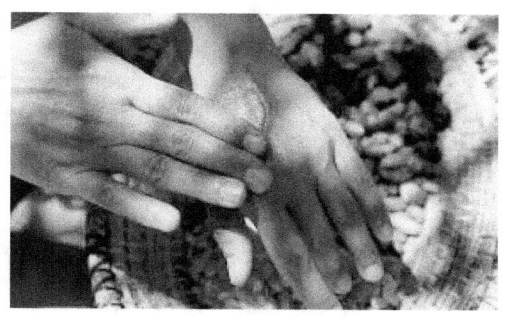

ONE OF THE RAREST AND MOST UNIQUE OILS IN THE WORLD

The Argan tree is known all through the Berber state in Morocco as the "Tree of Life." Pure Argan oil is produced using the parts of the nuts from argan trees.

Today, Argan trees become only in the semi-betray soil of the Arganeraie Biosphere Reserve. Because of this little and particular developing region, the trees are secured by the United Nations Educational, Scientific and Cultural Organization (UNESCO) and unadulterated Argan oil is one of the rarest on the planet.

The unadulterated Argan oil industry is nearly as special as the oil itself. All Argan sold today originates from cooperatives worked by Moroccan ladies, and the cooperatives share benefits among the neighborhood ladies of the Berber tribe. The cash goes toward medicinal services and instruction, and additionally other acts of kindness. For instance, Argan oil benefits built up a biological system reforestation extend so that Argan can be sourced scrupulously and the supply won't run out.

Significantly more amazing is that incomes from unadulterated Argan oil deals are accounted for to nourish 10% of the Moroccan populace.

SUPERB FOR SKIN, HAIR, AND NAILS… AND THE WORLD

"Late logical studies have demonstrated advantages of Argan oil has antimicrobial properties, and can be utilized as a part of treating harmed skin and irritation," said Majda Alaoui Sosso, executive of one of Morocco's oil cooperatives.

This is to a limited extent because of Argan oil's rich stores of key unsaturated fats, or EFAs, which bolster the wellbeing and excellence of skin and hair (while likewise, when taken inside, boosting heart and cerebrum wellbeing and directing hormone levels and other basic capacities).

Immaculate Argan oil is effortlessly retained, and it manages the pH adjust of the skin, which thus ensures against sun presentation and other harm. It likewise lessens skin irritation and accordingly controls and switch skin issue, for example, dermatitis and psoriasis while additionally decreasing scars.

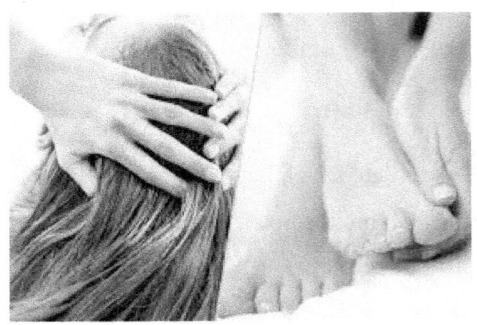

Immaculate Argan oil's demonstrated and watched benefits for hair, skin, and nails are broad, and incorporate, to give some examples...

• Dry Skin: Nourishes and saturates dry, textured, flaky skin and secures against contamination.

• Oily Skin: Regulates sebum creation to keep the skin's characteristic oils at a sound level. With standard utilize, the skin will not look anymore or feel sleek.

• Irritated/Itchy Skin: Protects skin from allergens that may bring about irritation.

• Acne: Controls overproduction of skin break out bringing on sebum and relieves the irritation achieved by skin inflammation; likewise keeps the appalling scars skin inflammation can desert.

• Aging: Stimulates reestablishment of skin cells and helps versatility while smoothing wrinkles and lines.

• Sun Damage Rich in cancer prevention agents that shield cells from UV light.

• Eczema and Psoriasis: Helps mitigate incendiary side effects connected with psoriasis. Additionally addresses resistance issues and sensitivities that trigger skin inflammation indications.

• Hair: Repairs harmed hair. Saturates in a flash, and avoids split finishes while re-establishing sparkle. Builds hair development and controls, cure, and avoid dry and irritated scalp.

• Scalp: Keeps scalp solid and very much supported. A couple drops will ensure against dandruff. Keeps the foundations of the hair hydrated, secured, and very much fed.

• Nails: Keeps nails solid and sound and re-establishes regular sparkle while effectively determining weak nail issues.

REASONS YOU SHOULD BE USING ARGAN OIL ON YOUR FACE

At the point when the vast majority of us consider argan oil, we consider sparkly, bouncy hair. Yet, did you know it has astonishing advantages for your skin, as well? Here, Josie Maran, originator of Josie Maran beautifiers, lets you know every one of the motivations to get in on the pattern.

Argan oil is a natural antioxidant which helps to neutralize free radicals and protect the delicate soft tissues of the face and body. The oil is packed full of nutrients and essential fatty acids, including linoleic acid, and has been used for decades in the cosmetic and skin care industry.

One of the main benefits this oil can offer is a significant reduction in the signs of aging often seen in the skin. The oil works by revitalizing cell growth and can help to combat the damage caused by pollution, sun, stress, and smoking. It can help to smooth wrinkles on the face and body as well as softening the skin, and scientific studies have also shown an increase in skin elasticity and tightening when used regularly. It can help to cure various ailments as well as increase immunity against diseases and infections when taken internally. The healing properties found in it can be of tremendous benefit to those people with burn injuries while it relieves the pain in rheumatism and arthritis sufferers. It protects the cardiovascular system and is helpful in preventing several types of cancer.

Argan oil is very beneficial for skin and helps in keeping it hydrated and moisturized. This is bliss for women with oily skin, who are scared of using any other beauty products on their sensitive skin. It has been proved by clinical trials on several women that oil results in a huge improvement in skin elasticity in only 4 weeks. This effect of the oil helps in reduction of fine line and wrinkles from your face. The oil is also a great product for pregnant women. They can rub the oil in the areas that succumb to stretch marks. With the regular use of oil from the early pregnancy, the elasticity of skin will increase thereby reducing the onset of stretch marks in the later stage.

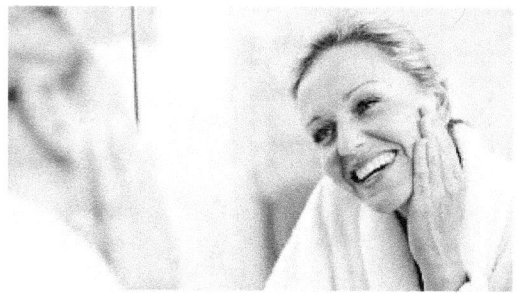

1. It's pressed with the well done.

Argan oil contains cancer prevention agents, vitamin E, and crucial unsaturated fats. "It's temperament's defensive, sustaining superfood for your skin," Maran says.

2. It will hydrate even the driest skin.

In case you're available for an exceptional lotion, look no more remote than Josie Maran's own 100% Pure Argan Oil. Does it seal in dampness, as well as shields skin from free radicals and other harming impacts from the outside environment (i.e. contamination).

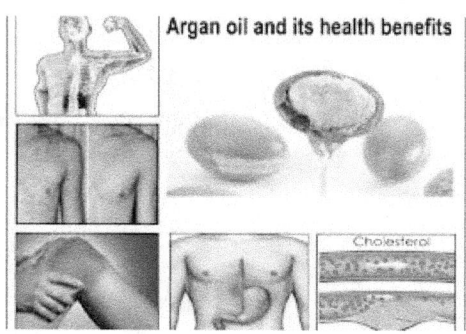

3. It won't oil up slick skin.

"It's incredible for slick skin since it attempts to really *control* oil creation," Maran says. "On the off chance that you deny your skin of oil, it regularly goes into overdrive and it can begin to overproduce oil. In the event that you utilize oil on your skin, it adjusts and kills your characteristic oil generation."

4. It won't stop up pores.

No doubt, we were agonized over putting unadulterated oil on our countenances as well. But since argan oil offsets your characteristic oil creation, it can really help with skin inflammation and flaws. Besides, "it's particularly tender on individuals with delicate skin conditions like dermatitis, psoriasis, and rosacea," Maran includes.

5. It's an against ager.

As though this oil isn't as of now doing what's needed, it can likewise be utilized as a hostile to maturing serum. Since it's a concentrated against oxidant, it will secure your skin's versatility.

6. It can be utilized night and day.

"Argan oil is sufficiently light to use as a day by day lotion and hydrating enough to use as an overnight treatment," Maran says. Two items at the cost of one? Sold.

11 MIRACLE BENEFITS OF ARGAN OIL FOR SKIN, HAIR & HEALTH

The fame of Argan Oil has detonated since the numerous astonishing medical advantages offered by this 'supernatural occurrence oil' have been made open. Icy squeezed from the product of the Moroccan Argan Tree (Argania spinosa) Argan Oil can be utilized both cosmetically and culinary to enhance everything from skin appearance to heart wellbeing.

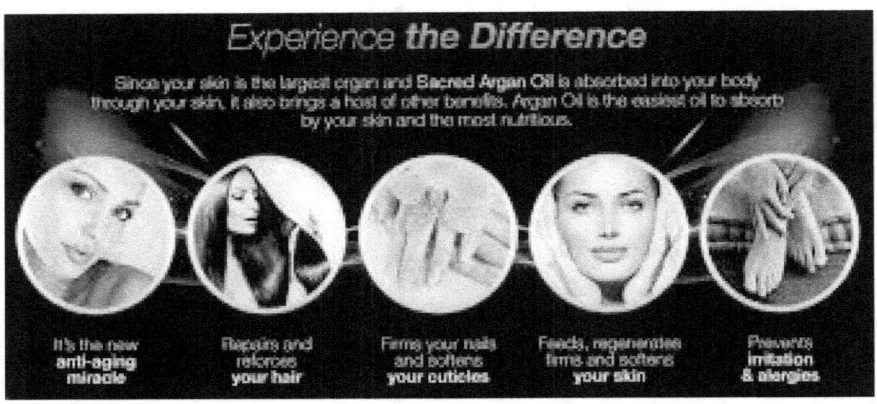

1. Recuperates Skin Ailments

The triterpenoids actually found in Argan oil offer stunning medical advantages for skin including the capacity to stunt the development of warts, treat a few types of dermatitis, separate tumorous skin cells, and blur scars. Likewise, the cell reinforcements and unsaturated fats found in Argan oil may likewise help with the treatment of gentle skin break out and with the recuperating of skin break out related scarring.

2. Diminishes Premature Aging

Argan oil is involved around 80% unsaturated fats which work marvels to delete indications of untimely maturing. Normal utilization of Argan oil has been demonstrated to diminish the profundity and seriousness of wrinkles, and also to blur age spots by re-establishing skin's energetic flexibility and by expanding the regenerative rate of solid skin cells.

3. Ensures Against Environmental Damage

Hostile to oxidants in Argan oil secure skin, hair, and nails from harm created by UV radiation. Applying Argan oil to UV harmed skin can really blur sun spots and recuperate the dry rough skin that outcomes from over-introduction to UV by advancing the recovery of sound cells.

4. Brings down Cholesterol

Culinary-review Argan oil, when utilized as a substitute for different less-solid oils in the eating routine can bring down awful cholesterol levels. The one of a kind mix of plant sterols found in Argan Oil – schottenol and spinasterol – really obstruct the ingestion of terrible cholesterol from inside the intestinal tract.

5. Mitigating

Flavonoids display in Argan oil has capable mitigating properties which can be utilized to treat both outer and inside issues. For alleviation from sore muscles and joints, knead a couple drops of unadulterated Argan oil into your skin over the influenced range. The individuals who battle with Polycystic Ovarian Syndrome, unnecessary weight increase, poor assimilation, or bladder issues may likewise profit significantly from the inward mitigating capacities of culinary-review Argan oil.

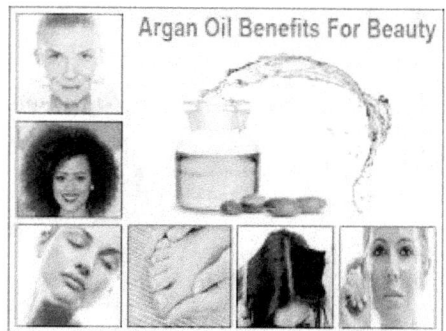

6. Helps Digestion

Culinary review Argan oil added to nourishment expands pepsin fixation in the body's gastric juices, in this way enhancing assimilation. Better absorption implies more vitality, less craving, enhanced weight reduction and an inside and out more advantageous body.

7. Battles Chronic Illness

There have been numerous studies with respect to the capacity of Argan oil to battle growth and different illnesses. Hostile to oxidants in Argan oil shield skin from free-radicals which can prompt to skin tumor. There have likewise been studies on the mending force of Argan oil against colon and bladder diseases, prostate malignancy, and dangerous developments all through the body which may come about because of contamination or aggravation.

8. Averts Stretch Marks

The recuperating force of Argan oil on skin doesn't stop with maturing and tumor medicines. This supernatural occurrence oil can likewise be utilized to keep extend marks from pregnancy, pubescent development of hips and mammaries, or from fast weight pick up by softening and fortifying skin.

9. Repairs Split Ends

At the point when connected to hair, Argan oil counteracts drying and ecological harm by covering the hair shaft. The oil seals in dampness and smooths fly-away, making hair more sensible and less inclined to breakage from brushing and styling. Argan oil can likewise seal in colorants, for example, henna and amla, expanding the time span between colorings. Rich in Vitamin-E, Argan oil supports hair, repairing split finishes, and builds hair's sparkle and general sound appearance.

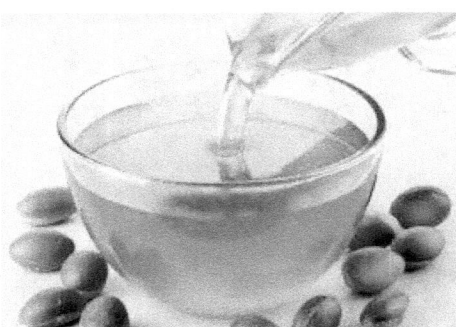

10. Fortifies Nails

At the point when connected to the fingers and toes, Argan oil advances more grounded, more advantageous nails normally with abnormal amounts of Vitamin-E. The counter bacterial and calming characteristics of Argan oil may likewise battle off nail and skin diseases connected with poor nail wellbeing.

11. Enhances Skin Appearance

Notwithstanding for the individuals who don't have scarring, wrinkles, or some other skin disease, Argan oil can in any case make your skin delicate and supple. Saponins in Argan oil reactivate skin cells' capacity to recover, keeping your biggest and most imperative substantial organ solid and solid.

While there are numerous less expensive Argan oil "mixed drinks" accessible in the wellbeing and excellence advertise which may have seriously decreased advantages to your wellbeing, 100% unadulterated Argan oil really is a supernatural occurrence oil to add to your common cure accumulation. Attempt this jug of Shea Terra Organics Argan Oil and see simply scraper superb this "supernatural occurrence oil" is!

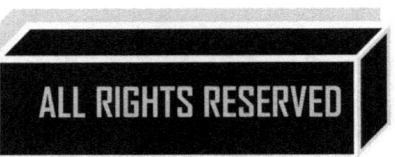